EAT LOOK WAY *Sexy*

THE
STRAIGHTFORWARD
GUIDE TO LOSING THE WEIGHT
AND HAVING THE CONFIDENCE
TO OWN WHO YOU ARE

DR. NADIA RIZZO, ND

Disclaimer notice

This is not intended to manage, diagnose, or treat any symptom or medical condition. You should always consult a licensed medical practitioner regarding your individual case prior to commencing any health intervention. This information is solely intended for informational and educational purposes.

Copyright © 2019 by Nadia Rizzo, ND.
All rights reserved. This book or any portion thereof may not be reproduced or used in any manner whatsoever without the express written permission of the publisher except for the use of brief quotations in a book review.

Publishing Services provided by Paper Raven Books
Printed in the United States of America
First Printing, 2019

Paperback ISBN: 978-1-9990959-0-1
Hardback ISBN: 978-1-9990959-1-8

TABLE OF CONTENTS

Preface	1
Introduction	3
Chapter 1: Protein	11
Chapter 2: The Gluten-Free Goddess	23
Chapter 3: Dump the Dairy	33
Chapter 4: Food Sensitivities	41
Chapter 5: Toxins, Stress, and Exercise	49
Chapter 6: The Bigger Picture	57
Acknowledgments	69

PREFACE

In June 2016, I gave birth to an amazing soul. I'm so blessed to be the mother of this beautiful boy who is gentle, sensitive, loving, affectionate, and nurturing. Less than one year after his birth, I found myself in the midst of a very unpleasant family court situation. During the chaos and negativity of this, I was supported immensely by my loved ones and the universe. What could have turned out to be a path of destruction, never-ending suffering, and sabotage wound up being one of the most transformational periods of my life. I was reconnected with my divine light, with God, and with my own heart. They say when the student is ready, the teacher appears. Books like *The Universe Has Your Back: Transform Fear to Faith* by Gabrielle Bernstein were appearing on my online feed. I felt compelled to read such books, and have found great power and comfort in the messages that lie within those pages. My son would nap and I'd sit next to him, in our dimmed room, reading, word after word, page after page. Praying. Trusting. Trying to let go of my vision and accept a reality greater than I could have ever dreamed. During all this, I realized I had also come into alignment physically. I was energized, amidst the emotional chaos of family court, I was fit, but more importantly, I was comfortable and confident in my own body. I wasn't even thinking about body image or such goals but focused on the spiritual path of higher learning. What I have learned is that when we are living in alignment with our true selves, our Creator, in divine spirit, everything else aligns as such.

I wrote this book because when I look back, I had a lot of "aha" moments—sure, with the things I was doing nutritionally but even more so with the lessons I learned along the way. This isn't a lecture. When I read this work, I have flashbacks to those days, sitting next to my sleeping baby boy, divinely placed books in hand, and spirit leading the way. I always say to my dear friend Dr. Laura Belus, ND that I don't want to just give health information, I want people to feel like they're sitting having tea and sharing conversation and higher truths with an actual person—sharing a divinely led connection. This isn't just storytelling. It's a sharing of the soul.

INTRODUCTION

Sexy isn't a number. It's not your dress size, how tall you are, how small your waist is, or even how big your boobs are. It's also not just a feeling or just confidence. It's more than all of those things. Some of us think that sexy is something we have to create, something we have to put on or consume from a bottle. It's not. It's something we all innately have within us; it's just something we have to tap into. Sexy is an **inner knowingness, an internal state of being.** Sexy is something that any of us can access at any time. Sexy is not something you have to *be*, it's just something you have to *remember*.

As a Naturopathic Doctor, I have supported countless patients in their journeys to feel their best, and many of them come to me for help with the motivation to lose weight. They want to be fit, and they want to feel sexy. But what exactly does it mean to be sexy?

Sexy is knowing who you are, owning your power, and living life from a place of eternal divine light. The false belief that you are separate from that divine source (creator/God/whatever label you want to use) is the reason for all suffering, the reason you feel disconnected.[1] When we tap into being connected to our true selves, our souls, and integrate that connection with our physical being, this human experience becomes far less scary, far less uncomfortable, and far easier to be embraced as an opportunity for growth and ascension of the soul.

The Lesson of Discernment

I just had to let someone go, and it hurt like hell. I cried. He doesn't know that I cried, but I did. He wasn't the father of my son, and he wasn't a fiancé (I've had two, you know, and I'm only having one more). Leaving those relationships was relatively easy (relatively, in comparison to this). Here is the thing. When we make decisions that WE KNOW are in alignment, our soul is able to ascend to higher processes, which is what we came here to do. But we don't want to remain here. We want to reach enlightenment, so we need to proceed forward, upward, onward, beyond all space and time. **When we make decisions that are in alignment with our soul's highest path, everything aligns, which brings about physical changes to our bodies, even losing weight.** My first serious relationship was with an amazing man, God bless him. He was gold of the earth, treated me

---
1 Helen Schucman, *A Course in Miracles* (Mill Valley, CA: Foundation for Inner Peace, 2007)

Introduction

like a freaking queen, and was my best friend. I won't get into why that wedding got cancelled. We loved each other, and I am certain we always will. I lost about 15 pounds when I released that first serious relationship. I went down a dress size without trying to lose weight, and it occurred to me that the body responds cellularly to soul alignment. The second serious relationship was with the father of my son, and let's just leave it at that. I shifted majorly after releasing that relationship, but by this time I had also learned other ways to help that shift, which I will share in this book with you. And finally, there is this relationship, the one I had to release. It was hard. Really hard. However, I know it's in the highest good for him and for me. We didn't formally label our relationship, but this long, dragged-out process of "getting to know each other" again after 12 years had run its course. So here I am, at my home desk with a barrel of gummy bears open, chocolate already down the hatch, and a beet juice in hand, because you know that will negate it all (sarcasm).

Ok, so let's just get to the point, please: **when you live your life in alignment with what your soul needs to be doing to ascend to higher levels of being, your body will respond.** It's like that thing (what the heck is it called?) where you pull the ball on the end and let it fall, causing the middle balls to vibrate so much that the last ball on the other side goes flying without the middle balls moving. It's like that. The vibration is carried, and because we are still here in the physical, our bodies are affected. So, when we live in a low vibration state—hate ourselves, blame ourselves, fail to grow and learn—and when we live seeking to fulfill our highest truth and make decisions in alignment with said highest truth, our bodies respond. You can imagine how vastly different each response would be between living in the hating state versus living in the loving state. Nothing goes unnoticed. Energy surrounds us all, and we have the power to co-create our lives, circumstances, living, jobs, money, love, relationships, kinships, travels, business, and, yes, even OUR BODIES.

So, here I am. I didn't expect to start with that, and I bet you didn't expect it either. I was thinking I'd just sneak it in there somewhere, but you know what, it's exactly where it needs to be: upfront, in our faces. If there is only ONE THING you take from this book, and even if you stop reading right now, I hope you are reminded of what you already know on another level: our souls are who we are. We are divine light, we are energetic frequencies, and when we set the intention to live our lives with good favor, kindness, and the benefit of the highest good being fulfilled, we live our truth, and our bodies respond. It won't even be about the weight anymore; the weight is a by-product of what is going on at another level. I am here to tell you how we can set the intention to live our lives in alignment with our personal truth and, in turn, see how our bodies react for the better.

From Projection to Living in Your Light

I recently found out that patients of other practitioners in my clinic have been commenting on my photo on my business card. Apparently, they have been saying that I am "pushing out my breasts." First of all, if a female does have large breasts, where does one expect her to put them?

Introduction

Hunch over and wrap her arms around them? (I'm getting slightly triggered here.) Second of all, I was pregnant in this photo, and during my pregnancy, my bra cup size was a DD. My photographer edited the photo so that I could use it long term for business. Well, it's certainly gaining me quite the attention. Ha! Interestingly, it's not men making these comments, it's WOMEN! At first, I was seriously taken aback. I felt judged, criticized, and kind of down to be honest. But as I reflected further, I recalled a time when I, too, used to pass such judgement on other females. If a woman was wearing something tight, I would think, "Well, she's a slut" or if she had a very toned butt, I would wonder, "Do you really have to wear such tight pants?" All this shit is a projection of the person's own insecurity. I was judgmental, because I was uncomfortable in my own body. The other day, a family member commented on my short shorts, and my internal reply was: "Do NOT shame me for being comfortable in my body simply because you are uncomfortable in yours." I can connect these dots, because I used to be SO judgmental of other females and their bodies before I was ever comfortable in mine. Now, I celebrate their beauty. I admire them. I bless them. I sometimes still get triggered, but my perspective and healing around this has shifted majorly. It's not about a certain dress size or bra size or how toned your buttocks are. It really comes down to being COMFORTABLE in your own skin. I am taking a moment now before starting my clinic shift to send gold healing light to all those who are experiencing discomfort, sadness, inadequacy, and frustration when it comes to their body. It doesn't have to be that way, and I am here to show you that.

The Notion of Wanting to Feel Sexy

I remember when I posted in a mom's group about the potential title for this book. I already knew it was going to be called *Eat Your Way Sexy*, and for some reason, in that moment, I felt the need to seek validation from the masses online. So, I posted two title options in this mom's group chat: 1. *Eat Your Way Sexy* and 2. *The Mom's Eating Plan*. I was set on the name for the book, but one mom's comment made me pause. She said, "Sexy? I am not trying to feel sexy! I am busy and tired. I just want more energy. Are you even a mom?" I laughed, felt bad for her, and felt a bit outraged all at the same time. First of all, YES, I AM A MOM. Who posts in a mom's group about something they are trying to cater to a mom population without even being a mom? Secondly, well, of course you want energy, and—newsflash!—feeling exhausted and walking around like a zombie is not sexy. Having energy is part of embodying sexiness. Thirdly, BULLSHIT! Bullshit that you don't want to feel sexy. I don't care what age you are, how many kids you have, if you are married, single, or divorced. EVERY WOMAN wants to feel sexy. It is not for someone else but for OURSELVES. I don't know what happened that had you repress, shove down, ignore, neglect, pretend to believe, or even actually believe that being sexy isn't an option for you, because it's absolutely FUCKING NOT TRUE. That is bullshit, and don't you dare believe it for one second.

I feel like this especially happens postpartum, when women start to say to themselves, "Well, I'm a mom and wanting energy is all I can ask for right now. Feeling sexy in my own skin doesn't matter." What is this shit? Postpartum is a peak time when a woman should honor all her body has just done, and it is an absolute fucking golden opportunity for us to begin feeling confident, sexy, and powerful in our own skin. You just brought another human being into the world and acted as a gateway between the spiritual and physical realms. You just brought about CREATION in one of its purest, most loving, and most beautiful forms. YEAH, SWEETHEART, YOU ARE FUCKING SEXY. (I'm like waving my arms around as these words come out because I cannot shout this loudly enough.) You have permission to be all of these things. You can be the mom, you can be energetic, and you can still be a fucking sexy woman who steps into her light, lives in her power, and is honored, respected, loved, and cherished for all that you are, simply because you exist. You don't have to do or say anything. This is not something you "earn." It's yours, and no matter what your circumstances are, you can own it, and nobody can take away that power from you. You are beautiful, you are worthy, you are loved, and, of course, YOU ARE SEXY.

Medical Considerations

Before we jump into how to eat your way sexy, it's important to note any medical investigations that should be considered. These factors could impact your health journey at large, including weight loss. Whether weight loss is a new goal for you, or it is something you have felt challenged with for a longer time, there are several medical things you should get clear on when it comes to weight loss, as several factors can be playing a part. Always follow up with your medical practitioner about your individual case. Some important things to rule out and manage include:

- Thyroid imbalances
  Please make sure a FULL comprehensive thyroid panel is run. That means not just your TSH but also your T3, T4, and thyroid antibody counts.
- Cortisol imbalances
  This is especially important for morning cortisol.
- Iron levels
- All sex hormones
- Pathologies of any sort
- Medications and side effects
- Nutrient depletions
- Natural health products and side effects

CHAPTER 1: PROTEIN

Oh, where to begin? Protein is one of THE MOST important things you could learn about in this book. Ok, I might say that about nearly every topic, but it's really true. Protein is important for so many functions of the body, including immunity and blood sugar stabilization, which can affect mood, energy, and even hormones. Oh, and did I mention weight loss? Here's the thing you need to understand: when we eat carbohydrates, they turn into sugar in the bloodstream. Now, when we eat protein WITH the carbs, it helps to slow the release of sugar into the bloodstream. This is important, because when our blood sugar goes up all of a sudden, guess what? It crashes "all of a sudden," too. Blood sugar going up and down makes our mood and energy go up and down and can seriously start to screw with our hormones if it goes on for long enough. What people tend to disregard is that insulin (the hormone needed to help us take glucose or sugar into the cell) is just that: a HORMONE.

It's signaled by blood sugar levels, so when our blood sugar goes up, insulin gets told to do its thing and take the sugar into the cells of the body. However, when we eat more glucose or sugar, our body now needs to pump out more insulin because, well, obviously you need more for the job since there's more sugar to take in.

Let's think about it another way. A simpler way. If blood sugar is a bunch of tiny packages and insulin is the delivery truck that needs to get these packages to the cell, the more packages (blood sugar) we have, the more delivery trucks (insulin) we need, right? Makes sense. But, what happens over time is that if we are constantly overdoing it with spiking our blood sugar, we may develop what is called "insulin resistance." This may sound familiar to you if you know someone who has type 2 diabetes. It is actually also commonly the case with polycystic ovarian syndrome (PCOS). Now, although this would take time to manifest and isn't going to happen from eating one huge dose of cupcakes, the point is that screwing with our blood sugar can screw with our hormones. Allowing our blood sugar to spike like that isn't a good (or comfortable) habit to have, because it's like making things work in overdrive.

So, what does this mean, Dr. Rizzo? Can I NEVER eat cupcakes? Hell to the no, girl. See, if I told you that you could never eat a treat, that means that I would have to live by that same rule, and I am just not up for that. My treat will be gluten- and dairy-free and free of my food sensitivities (more on that later), but a treat it still shall be. The trick I have up my sleeve is that when I do eat carbs, I eat them with protein (mmm, steak). See, when we eat carbs with ENOUGH protein, the blood sugar increases very slowly without spiking, and we are less likely to crash. We are also less likely to get hungry all of a sudden or feel like we need to pop a chocolate bar to keep going. All good things, right?

So that is the BIGGEST takeaway on protein: it helps us regulate our blood sugar. However, I don't want you to go and eat a ton of cupcakes with a steak every day. Let's not be extreme here. It's great to have the trick up your sleeve, but I also want you to understand that it's important to know how much protein you should be getting and how many carbs are too many. You may already know this, but carbs are not just bread, rice, starches, and potatoes. Carbs are in fruit and vegetables, too. Use the reference guide on page 14 to approximate protein and carbohydrate counts for common foods.

Protein Sources

Animal Protein Sources	Plant-Based Protein Sources
Red Meat (Pork, Beef, Veal)	Legumes (Lentils, Chickpeas)
Poultry (Chicken, Turkey)	Beans
Lamb	Quinoa
Fish	Peas
Dairy (Cheese, Milk)	Nuts, Nut Butters, & Seeds
Eggs	Hemp
Whey	Chia

The Vegan Protein Masterlist

	Amount	Protein (grams)	Carbohydrates (grams)
Chia	1 TBSP	= 3g protein =	6g carbs
Kidney Beans	1/2 CUP *cooked	= 8g protein =	18g carbs
Navy beans	1/2 CUP *cooked	= 7g protein =	20g carbs
Lentils	1/2 CUP *raw	= 25 g protein =	58g carbs
Chickpeas	1/2 CUP *cooked	= 7g protein =	23g carbs
Hemp Shells	3 TBSP	= 10g protein =	1g carbs
Almonds (raw)	1/4 CUP	= 8g protein =	7g carbs
Peanut Butter	2 TBSP	= 7g protein =	7g carb
Peas	3/4 CUP *frozen	= 5g protein =	14g carbs
Quinoa	1/4 CUP	= 6g protein =	29g carbs
Vegan All-in-One Protein Powder	1 SCOOP	= 15-20 g protein =	11-13g carbs

Animal Versus Vegan Protein Sources

I must start this off by saying that I am not here to challenge you on any of your beliefs. I know people who eat a vegan-based diet for a variety of reasons, and I respect everyone's free will to eat as they so choose. However, I am also here to educate you. It is my responsibility to point out that this is a book focused on weight loss, and having a vegan diet whilst trying to lose weight can be extremely challenging. The reason is obvious when you take a look at the reference guide on vegan sources of protein and their parallel carbohydrate doses on page 14. By the time we eat enough of a vegan source to get enough protein, we have also consumed a ton of carbs. In a nutshell (no pun intended), vegan sources of protein tend to be quite carbohydrate heavy. Remember, carbs can spike our blood sugar, and heavy carb loads can crash our energy. Some vegan protein powders are formulated to accommodate this, which is great. Meaning, they are compounded to be low carb but high protein. I actually use vegan protein powder for my shakes, because whey doesn't sit well with me, but I still consume animal protein as a large part of my diet.

Animal Protein Sources

If you are going to consume animal protein, it is always best for it to be organic. Take into consideration how that animal was raised, because, girl, if it had extra hormones getting pumped into its body, let's not even pretend that shit isn't getting transferred to us when we eat it. I always aim for grass-fed beef and animals that were raised consciously, kindly, and antibiotic-free. Know your sources. If you feel overwhelmed, just start with one thing. Maybe you don't switch all of your chicken, but you just switch your beef. This is not an overnight change. Step-by-step will get you there and KEEP you there, honey. Extreme fast changes tend to lead to crash and burn (*thinks of how this has also been true for personal relationships* :). #LIVEANDLEARN

The Vegan Weight Loss Dance

The issue with many vegan sources is, while they are great sources of vegan protein, they are relatively carb heavy. Let's break it down. Carbs turn into sugar in the blood. We don't want too much sugar. As such, it's good to limit our intake of carbs. A general guideline is a maximum of approximately 30 grams of carbs per day and 10 grams of carbs per serving. If you were to take in the full 30 grams at once, that would just likely spike the blood sugar right up, so it's better to spread it out. With many legumes, to get enough protein to suffice for a serving, you also have to take in a high carb count, and now we do this dance. For example, 1/2 cup of cooked chickpeas renders less than 10 grams of protein but has over 20 grams of carbs! So, it doesn't meet the minimum amount of protein per serving and exceeds the maximum recommended serving of carbs. Such is the struggle of being a master at vegan eating if you want to lose weight. I am a glass-is-half-full type of person, but I am not going to sugarcoat it: vegan eating mixed with weight loss goals is freaking difficult, partially because of the dance between protein and carbs.

Chapter 1: Protein

Nutrient Deficiencies and the Vegan Diet

Vegan protein has a void of vitamin B12, also known as cobalamin, which comes from animal sources. In addition to vitamin B12, a vegan diet can make things very difficult when it comes to increasing our iron stores in the body. The reality is that animal sources of iron are much more readily absorbed than vegan sources of iron. I can already energetically feel the voices raising, the arms waving, and the protesters marching. Please allow me to remind you I am here to educate you, not to fight you. I am here to support you, not to convert you. The fact of the matter is that even those vegan sources of iron that are absorbed quite nicely can be stopped by many things. There are little things called "oxalates" that are basically big stop signs for iron. These oxalates are present in food sources like grains, such as barley, and even in some vegetables like spinach. So, when you eat your beets and kale salad with your grains at lunch, you are basically ingesting a stop sign for absorption of iron from your vegan iron foods. Yes, it's true that oxalates can actually stop the absorption of iron from vegan foods.

I can feel you thinking, "Ahhhh, that makes sense now." I can already feel the dots connecting and the guards coming down. You might be wondering why nobody has told you that before. Let me tell you that I am lucky that I even learned that fact. I was sitting in a Starbucks studying for my naturopathic medical board exams, and I remember reading that in the review material. I was like, "DAMN, how did I miss this?" Sometimes it doesn't get taught, and sometimes we forget things. But, 100% of the time practitioners and doctors are HUMAN BEINGS LIKE YOU, and it is impossible for any human being to know absolutely every single detail about every little thing even when we have studied the subject for a decade or more. The fact that I even remember (total flashback to sitting in that cafe right now) reading that page and having that "WHOA" moment was **divinely placed** because I was meant to be the messenger to bring this to all of you. I know that even just realizing that fact that oxalates can block the absorption of iron from vegan food sources will change the quality of so many of your lives. Let's all just take a moment and thank divine timing right now.

Here is a list of some main foods that contain oxalates, but please note this is NOT fully inclusive:

- Barley
- Beets
- Peanuts
- Spinach
- Yellow and white potatoes

Protein and Your Energy

As we have already established, protein is so important for blood sugar regulation. When we eat simple carbohydrates (i.e., a piece of bread), we get this surge of energy, often followed by a huge energy crash. This is your blood sugar spiking. Simple carbs and high glycemic index foods turn into sugar quickly and enter the bloodstream rapidly. They cause an energetic high only to be followed by a much undesired energetic low.

The more we do this, the more our body has to work overtime to manage the situation. Let's talk about insulin. To be clear, insulin is a hormone made by the pancreas that acts like a little taxi, carrying sugar from the bloodstream into the cells to be used for energetic processes in the body. What happens when we overdo it constantly with the high sugar/glycemic index foods? We build up tolerance, and just like someone struggling with an addiction who requires more and more of a substance to get that same high, we need more and more insulin to get that glucose (sugar) into the cells. This puts extra pressure on our bodies, leads to poor blood sugar management over time, resulting in weight gain and screwing with other hormones in the long run. So, what to do? When you eat carbs, never eat them alone and always add protein. It slows the release and conversion of carbs to sugar into the bloodstream and helps us avoid spikes in our blood sugar.

How much protein is enough? It's generally based on weight but is also affected by physical activity and any physical diagnosis that one may have, such as kidney disease. As a general guideline (key word: GENERAL), this calculation is helpful: **0.6g/kg of body weight.**[2]

So, if someone weighs 200 pounds, we have to convert that into kg (divide by 2.2): 200/2.2 = 90.9kg x 0.6g/kg = 54.54g. So, we can say that as a general guideline, someone who weighs 200 pounds should aim to intake a minimum of approximately 55 grams of protein a day. To reiterate, this is general. If someone has certain fitness habits or medical conditions or is on certain medications, this number may not be accurate. Hence, it's important to work together with

---

[2] Prousky, Jonathan, *Textbook of Integrative Clinical Nutrition* (Toronto, Ontario: CCNM Press, 2012)

a qualified practitioner one-on-one to evaluate your specific case and make an appropriate plan for you.

How many carbs are too many? If someone is dealing with blood sugar dysregulation or insulin issues, a general guideline is approximately 10g carbs maximum per serving and approximately 30g max per day. I even try to follow this myself most of the time, but there are certainly times when I consume greater amounts. Please note that these general numbers may change based on your individual circumstances and, as such, it is always important to get your case analyzed by a qualified medical professional. It is possible that blood sugar levels can go too low, and this would be an issue too if you are dealing with a blood sugar related pathology.

Snacking

If you are a snacker, make sure you are adding extra protein to your carby snack. Fruit is a great example. Pair apples and pears with an organic nut butter. Add hemp or chia seeds on top of a banana. Add hemp to soups, smoothies, salads, and pretty much any food you can imagine. The addition of the protein to the carb source will help slow and steady the release of the carbs into the blood in the form of sugar. This will aid in the stabilization of blood sugar as opposed to a quick spike in blood sugar levels.

Protein helps us stay fuller longer. Eating without protein is like asking for a quick energy high followed by a deep energy crash that's lower than low and draining. Protein is also important for the function of our cells. Protein forms muscles, tendons, and organs, assists in neurocognitive functions, and—given the role protein plays when it comes to blood sugar—it can even affect our mood! **A diet deficient in protein is a recipe for feeling like shit.** Hey, I am just going to be real with you. It is what it is.

Beauty Meets Protein

If you need a vanity point here to help push yourself with the protein bit of this whole equation, here it is: our hair is actually made of protein. How can we expect to build something stronger, thicker, and fuller if we aren't giving it the building blocks to do the job? It's like saying you want to build a house but you don't have any bricks. Protein is what hair is made of, and we need to be taking it in through our diet if we expect to improve our hair. We should note here that hair thinning can be due to hormones, low iron, and other factors as well but protein can play a major role for the above reasons.

I think back to my earlier postpartum days and how I started upping my protein. You know what I got from it? More energy, less crankiness, great hair, and a body I was more comfortable in after having a baby than I had EVER been before. Girl, if you put down this book right now and never pick it up again (but obviously you won't do that), I know that this section on protein will have changed your life. It's the first chapter for a reason.

CHAPTER 2:
THE GLUTEN-FREE GODDESS

What is Gluten?

Gluten is basically a mixture of proteins that serve to make dough nice and chewy. (I'm literally salivating as I think back to my nonna's homemade puffy white bread dripping with butter). Maybe you've heard people of previous generations telling us how they ingested loads of wheat and they turned out "just fine." But it's worth considering that the wheat (and other gluten-containing grains) that they were ingesting in previous years may not be the same as the wheat we are ingesting today. Much of modern wheat is genetically modified, which means that the biochemical structure of it is very different from what it used to be. In addition, many harvests are sprayed with chemicals to help them sustain factors that threaten agriculture, such as insects and weather conditions. So, are we having a reaction to these grains themselves or to the biochemical engineering that has been done to it? Perhaps both.

It wasn't until I actually got myself off of gluten for a good few weeks that I realized how much better I felt. I wasn't so bloated all the time (although at the time I didn't realize how I was feeling was actually "bloatedness"). I lost a few pounds. But the most significant change was that I GOT MENTAL CLARITY! Man, I had no idea that I was living with brain fog. I didn't feel challenged at all when it came to concentration or academic tasks. But once I detoxed from gluten, I could not believe my potential and the level of mental clarity I had naturally achieved. It still amazes me as I look back and think of the transition, like a caterpillar turning into a butterfly.

Seriously. I just get so excited because I know that there are so many of you who are living with things that may seem normal to you but actually are just symptoms of your environment, food, etc. I know that once you detox yourself from your food sensitivities, you will gain advantages that you never even thought possible. So, as a start, I have attached a list of glutinous versus gluten-free grains for you to use as you embark on the path to discovering your full potential.

Chapter 2: The Gluten-Free Goddess

GLUTEN VS. GLUTEN FREE

GLUTEN	GLUTEN FREE
Wheat	Rice
• Semolina	• White
• Durum	• Wild
Whole wheat	• Basmati
Spelt	Buckwheat
Kamut	Millet
Barley	Amaranth
Panko	Quinoa
Udon	Sorghum
Orzo	Arrowroot
Bran	
Rye	
Pumpernickel	
Oats*	

*Note: Unless oats are certified gluten free, assume that they have GLUTEN! For the purposes of the elimination diet it may be best to stay away from all oats just to be as accurate as possible.

Celiac Versus Food Sensitivities

Celiac disease is an autoimmune condition that is genetic. Therefore, if nobody in your family has it, or if you do not have the gene, you cannot get it. This is not fully dependent on environmental factors; it has to be inherited. The cells of the intestines are literally attacking themselves whenever the gluten comes into the system. These individuals get terrible abdominal pain, unpleasant bowel disturbances, and large flare-ups of inflammation in their bodies whenever they come into contact with gluten. Food sensitivities, on the other hand, are not necessarily genetic. They have more to do with our bodies simply not accepting a food as friendly, or the bioengineering that has been done to a food. Eating foods that we are sensitive to can induce inflammatory reactions in our bodies, and inflammation isn't exactly an environment conducive to health. Read on to get the scoop on food sensitivities in further detail.

Did you ever think that a hidden food sensitivity could be the reason you are feeling so crappy?

I hate diets. I don't believe in them. But there is one diet that I've done several times myself that is used as a medical detective tool and actually has the potential to promise long-term, sustainable results. This diet is the elimination diet.

What is the elimination diet?

The elimination diet is a means to figure out if one is sensitive to certain foods. In a nutshell, it is approximately three to four weeks of eating clean and eliminating a list of foods that could be inducing inflammation and leading to symptoms such as bloating, joint pain, fatigue, brain fog, etc. Then there is a phase of reintroduction (the fun part), where eliminated foods are reintroduced in a very systematic process to see if any symptoms are experienced.

Wouldn't I get the symptoms now? Why eliminate and reintroduce?

Good question. Well, my friends, the truth is that when we are exposing our precious bodies to these potential triggers of feeling crappy on a regular basis, we just build a tolerant sense of "this is normal." We have no big hitter coming at us like a major headache out of nowhere (my lovely symptom upon reintroducing dairy) but rather a constant sense of "I feel sluggish" or "I feel bloated," for example. We need to rid our bodies of the junk, and then the effects will be made clear to us. It's like we lose the sense of what it feels like to function at high capacity, or we simply never knew it before at all.

What's the difference between a food sensitivity and a food allergy?

I'm so glad you asked. As one of my medical mentors put it to me when I was a student, "You have to understand the normal before you can understand the abnormal." So, let's take a brief stop at the basics. A reaction, whether that be an allergy or sensitivity, is basically our bodies' way of saying, "Hey, that's not normal" or "Shields up! This is harmful!" Our immune system is like an army, protecting us from harm.

Let's think of our antibodies as being little soldiers who are divided up into different camps.

Three main camps of soldiers:
IgE: think E for "emergency"
IgG: think G for "general"
IgA (primarily in the lungs and digestive tract): think A for "abdominal"

A food allergy is what causes anaphylaxis, a life-threatening situation where the throat begins to close. This type of reaction is the reason so many kids carry EpiPens with them and schools do not allow peanuts. This has to do with a release of IgE. That is NOT what we are talking about when referring to a food sensitivity. A food sensitivity has to do with the workings of IgG and IgA. That is, when we eat a food that we are sensitive to, it causes a spike in IgG and/or potentially IgA, which can translate into a boatload of inflammation.

What's inflammation got to do with it? ("Got to do, got to do with it." Anyone? Come on guys…)

Well, my friends, to keep things simple and sweet, inflammation can make our bodies feel pretty crappy. If you already have an inflammatory condition, like arthritis for example, it is possible that this can aggravate and flare up your pain. Inflammation can also be sneaky. Let's take my own case for example. I had no idea that my once-upon-a-time hidden food sensitivity of potato (organic and baked) was causing my bloating, unhappy tummy, and fatigue. When I eat that thing, even if it's not fried, boy do I regret it. It's "see ya later skinny jeans and hello brain fog" until the reaction subsides days later.

Why do an elimination diet?

You might do one if you suspect you are having a reaction to certain foods, or—and this is far more common—if you have tried many other things and still cannot figure out why you are feeling the way you are feeling (bloated, lethargic, mental fogginess, skin stuff—sound familiar?).

Who should not do an elimination diet?

If you are pregnant or breastfeeding, it is best NOT to do an elimination diet. If you have a medical condition, always check with your medical doctor prior to beginning any intervention.

My First Elimination Diet Experience

I remember the first time I did an elimination diet. Oh my goodness! The beginning was so challenging. I remember bawling my eyes out at my parents' kitchen table, because I was so overwhelmed and frustrated. I felt like I couldn't eat anything! But that's actually not true. You can eat a ton of stuff while on the elimination diet. The thing is, you need to have the right guidance and support to make it simplified. I mean, I survived my first one and ultimately improved my well-being, but the truth is I suffered through it, especially in the beginning. My practitioner basically said: "Ok, here are the lists of what you can and can't eat. See you in three weeks to walk you through the reintroduction phase." Insert dropped jaw emoticon here. Seriously. But I have to say that I am truly grateful for the experience, because it made me realize the importance of support and having the right guidance in order to get the best results. This epiphany for me in my first year of my naturopathic medical training sparked a passion inside of me. Long story short, this all fueled me to set up resources for anyone wanting help doing an elimination diet. I compiled grocery lists, recipes, checklists, preparation guides, tips to set you up for success, a private support group, and more. My recipes are super simple, too; many of you who know me by now would know that I am so into eating healthy but so NOT into cooking for hours on end.

If you want in on my online e-course, A Simplified Approach to the Elimination Diet, just go to www.nadiarizzo.com and click the contact tab. Send me a message, and I will get you the program registration details.

What REALLY fueled me to bring the information on food sensitivities forward was my postpartum experience. After having my baby, I stuck to avoiding my food sensitivities like my life depended on it and felt so much better. I did it because I needed the energy and just felt amazing in my own skin. I remember one day catching a glimpse of my reflection as I was running through the house, grabbing something in my son's room and simultaneously getting dressed whilst walking (#momlife). When I saw my bare abdomen in the mirror, I was slightly taken aback by how flat my stomach was. I hadn't avoided my food sensitivities because I wanted to be a Skinny Minnie; I was a single mom who needed every ounce of energy she could get, and I felt so good that I never wanted to go back to feeling shitty ever again. But when I looked in the mirror, I noticed for the first time what avoiding food sensitives had done for my belly fat, or what I thought was belly fat. But guess what? Girl, that wasn't belly fat. It was inflammation in the gut from eating foods I am sensitive to. I snapped a photo but never got the guts to post it. I was afraid people would say things or judge me, blah blah blah. But I did say to myself, "This will be part of my story one day." So here it is.

Eat Your Way Sexy

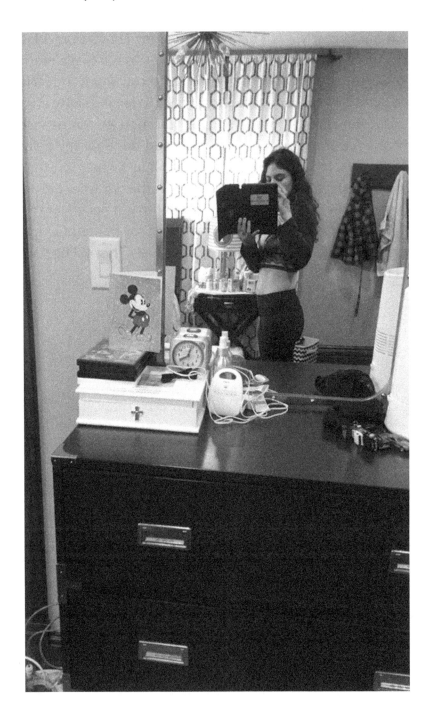

CHAPTER 3:
DUMP THE DAIRY

Going dairy-free is something that I like to try with those who have plateaued in their weight loss and have all of the other pieces of the puzzle in place. Often times, it's not simply "weight" but inflammation that we need to get rid of, causing us to plateau. It helps to think about the purpose of milk. We need to think about the purpose of milk as the life force that grows a calf into a cow. Much like human milk grows human babies, cow milk grows calves and makes them bigger. So, regardless of the fact that many of us lack the enzyme to break down milk properly (lactase enzyme), even those who can break down milk properly are still intaking a substance whose sole purpose from an evolutionary perspective is to grow baby cows into larger cows. I certainly wouldn't want to be taking something in that would balloon me up like a blimp when there is nothing in there that I can't get elsewhere. I can drink fortified nut milks, add supplements, and make sure the rest of my diet is clean and healthy. I really don't need to drink milk. Have I caught your attention? I thought so. Let's talk about the actual health potential of going dairy-free.

Lactose Versus Casein

The reason I can drink lactose-free milk and still feel sick is because my body doesn't just react to the lactose; it also reacts to the casein. Casein is a protein that our body can break down, but there are different forms of it. There are different kinds of casein proteins, which vary in their biochemical blueprint. The casein in cow milk is not necessarily the same as the casein in goat milk, which is why some people absolutely cannot drink cow milk, even if it is lactose-free, but can drink goat's milk without having to run to the toilet.

Cows, Goats, and Sheep

If you want to include dairy in your diet but it doesn't always sit well with you, I suggest you consider alternative sources. Now, we have already touched on the fact that goat's milk is made up of casein proteins that differ from those in cow's milk, so it may be a suitable option for you. However, sheep dairy sources tend to have higher protein levels. When I was pregnant and missing dairy, I would eat sheep yogurt. I didn't react to it quite like I would cow or goat, and I knew that it had the highest protein of all three sources, making it a double win. I remember drizzling some sweet balsamic on it, throwing in chia seeds, and enjoying that as a snack while I was preggers. Getting the extra protein made me feel better and was still a smarter snack than empty carbs like chips or muffins.

Traditional Chinese Medicine and Dairy

In Traditional Chinese Medicine (TCM), dairy is thought of as "dampness promoting." Dairy supports mucus production, so if there is a cold, respiratory condition, or flu hanging around, it's definitely not something I would want to be eating. Think of dampness like big white balls of gooey, semi-soft cheese. It blocks things and stuffs things up. From a TCM perspective, when things get stuffy or blocked, then the harmonious flow of energy (or qi) gets blocked or slowed down. Dampness is heavy and can slow the flow of qi, which is our life force and relates to many internal organ systems in the body.

This Shit Hides

Dairy hides in things we never would have thought contain dairy. Whey protein, for example, is a source of dairy. (One exception is butter, which I don't count, because it's basically just fat when it is boiled down.) Dairy can be mixed into so many things. Whenever I buy meatballs or want to order them at a restaurant, I always ask if there is dairy mixed into the batter. You might think you're just eating beef, but in my experience, more often than not you are also eating dairy. I remember being in the hospital after having my son and sending my then partner out to get food from an amazing Italian grocery store with a great hot table. He came back with meatballs, warm, covered in sauce. Mmm mmm. I looked at the label and saw "parmesan cheese." As an Italian, I should know that we put cheese in everything. So, when you think you're just ordering meat, you still need to clarify with the source that it's indeed dairy-free. Read the labels of the products you are buying, ask the chef, double and triple check. It can be annoying in the beginning, but once you get it down, it becomes second nature and you will learn where all of the dairy-free go-tos are in your area.

Dairy Alternatives

Now, often times people will ask me what they can eat instead of dairy. You don't necessarily need to replace your dairy. Just because you are ditching cheese doesn't mean you need to now find the most glorious "cheese-less cheese" vegan option. You can practice making dishes without dairy in them at all, even the fake dairy. My concern with many (not necessarily all, but many) "fake dairy" products is this: to remove the dairy or the fat, often times chemical crap needs to be added to keep the same consistency in the product (texture, etc.). Well, I don't like fake, and I definitely don't like eating chemicals. So, do I want to eat a "vegan cheese" if it means it's laden with a bunch of fake junk? No, I don't. At that point, I don't know what is worse: the fake crap or the potential inflammation from the real dairy. The point is that you can work around it.

Here are some dairy alternatives that I like using:

- **Milk** alternatives include almond, hemp, hazelnut, rice, and coconut milk. I love an iced coffee with a splash of nut milk and a dash of cinnamon. Some of these milks even come in chocolate!
- Speaking of **chocolate**, I won't tell you to ditch the chocolate but instead suggest you find good alternatives. There is a brand called Enjoy Life, which is dairy-free and soy-free (win-win in my book), and they make chocolate chips that are amazing. Raw Revolution is another great brand that I enjoy, and I can buy it online. Search and you shall find!
- I went crazy (in a good way) with vegan coconut **ice-cream** recipes one summer. It's so easy with my ice-cream maker. Canned, full-fat coconut milk works best. I searched online and found tons of free recipes. Alternatively, you can buy a dairy-free sorbet, but watch the sugar content.
- Instead of **whipped cream**, refrigerate a can of full-fat coconut milk overnight and turn it upside down in the morning (this is key). Keeping the can upside down, open it up from the bottom side. You can mix it lightly with a pinch of coconut sugar if you like and use as topping. Voila! Top with dairy-free chocolate shavings, if desired. (OMG who else is craving strawberries and banana with this right now? Can you taste it? I can.)
- Opt for hummus or mashed avocado **dips**. Or even mix them together (I love this combo). Half a crack-

er with hummus plus half a cracker with avocado equals an explosion of dairy-free goodness in my mouth! Are you salivating already?
- For **dressings,** hello pure extra virgin olive oil, freshly squeezed lemon juice, salt, and pepper! You can find flavored olive oils, too. Go nuts. I bet you'll never go back to the junk that comes in a plastic bottle once you find your olive oil muse.

Dairy Detox

Once you feel the benefit of eliminating a substance that inflames the heck out of your body, you always want more (don't we always want more of what makes us feel good?). Dairy detox is that way for me, so I created this free seven-day challenge for those who are looking for support with going dairy-free or just don't know where to start. Yes, it can seem daunting, but I promise that you can still eat a ton of things, and it's totally worth it. The way I feel when I stick to being dairy-free is so worth passing up the parmesan, and boy did I ever love parmesan (until I realized it was a huge contributor to the bloating). My favorite part of this challenge is on day four where I actually give you a guide on how to **eat out dairy-free** (hey girl, I know you're busy). EATING DAIRY-FREE DOES NOT MEAN BEING CONFINED AT HOME! Here is my quick guide for you when it comes to eating out dairy-free.

1. Appetizers. Always ask if they contain dairy. It hides in things you wouldn't expect.

2. Salads. No dressing. Request olive oil, lemon, salt, and pepper instead.

3. Soups. Ask if dairy is in them. So many are dairy-based and not broth-based.

4. Pasta. Avoid fancy sauces and opt for pure tomato basil sauce.

5. Meats. Clarify with the server how it's prepared. For example, my favorite dish—veal scaloppini—is made in a thin, dairy-free sauce at one restaurant location, but the same restaurant at a different location makes it with a dairy mushroom sauce. This caught me by surprise the first time it happened…a delicious but totally bloating surprise.

6. Pizza. Make sure there isn't any dairy in the dough! Always ask! Most sit-down restaurants will offer a dairy-free pizza. Ask for a pesto base without cheese or sauce and just add toppings. Chicken, olives, and sun-dried tomatoes go well with this. Oh, and artichokes! Mmm.

7. Coffee. Skip the cappuccino unless dairy-free milk, such as almond milk, is offered. Opt for tea or black coffee (coffee has more health benefits without milk anyway!).

8. Dessert. I'm skipping my childhood beloved ice-cream tartufo and sticking to dairy-free sorbet.

There you have it! You can still enjoy an amazing night out whilst ditching the dairy. You can sign up online for my free seven-day dairy detox at www.nadiarizzo.com/freebies.

CHAPTER 4: FOOD SENSITIVITIES

You Can't Do Anything with Information You Don't Have

The hidden key to unlocking the stubborn weight loss is recognizing that **it's not belly fat; it's inflammation in your gut from eating the foods you're sensitive to.** Let me point out that there is some repetition here. We briefly touched on food sensitivities already, but this chapter dives in even deeper. I also want to highlight that just because you may feel you aren't experiencing an actual physical reaction to your food sensitivities does NOT change the potential that an immune response is still at play on a biochemical level. Whether or not you tune into the feeling, your body is still responding and inflammation can still be raging. So, without further ado (and with some necessary repetition), let's jump in.

A food sensitivity is a food that your body doesn't "accept as friendly." When you eat this food, your body reacts in such a way that it mounts an immune response as a means of protecting itself. We have three major camps of antibodies when it comes to sensitivities: IgE, IgG, and IgA. First, let's just be clear that IgE is the antibody related to anaphylaxis. Think E for "emergency," as in life-threatening, in-need-of-an-EpiPen type of deal. This is NOT what we are talking about when discussing food sensitivities. A food sensitivity relates to two other main camps of antibodies: IgG and IgA. Think G for "general" and think A for "abdominal" (although IgA is also hanging out in the lungs, for the sake of our conversation let's stick with abdominal). When someone with an anaphylactic allergy eats a food they're allergic to, they have an immune reaction and the release of IgE can cause a life-threatening situation. Although food sensitivities are not instantaneously life threatening, much like an actual allergy, they cause an immune reaction and can induce an antibody increase. When we are talking about the antibodies related to food sensitivities, we are referring mainly to IgG and IgA. When we eat a food that we are sensitive to, these antibodies jump up and cause inflammation in the body. So, although ingesting foods we are sensitive to doesn't threaten our life, in that moment (just as a true allergy does), it induces an inflammatory reaction. A constant state of inflammation is not something anyone would want to live with, especially once you realize what this actually does to your body and mind.

If we have an antibody reaction and stop ingesting foods we are sensitive to, the reaction can subside within three days typically. However, symptoms can start to improve within

24 hours if properly managed. It's important to note that, although we can start to feel better, the immune reaction itself can still be at play. This is why when someone tells me they only eat the food they're sensitive to "sometimes," I break it down and explain that eating that food sometimes can still result in chronic problems. Let's use yogurt as an example, since dairy is definitely one of my personal food sensitivities. Even if you just eat yogurt twice a week, you can basically induce a constant state of inflammation. Remember, it can take approximately three days for the antibody reaction to resolve itself. So, if you eat that yogurt on Monday and the reaction chills out by Thursday, but then you eat that yogurt again on Thursday, you've just induced another immune reaction filled with inflammatory induction. So people tend to think that eating it "only twice a week" isn't a big deal and I can totally honor the good intention of limiting a food you are sensitive to, but as you can see, incorporating that food into a somewhat regular routine "sometimes" still messes us up. It's not worth it. Don't do it.

When we feel fat on most areas of our bodies (butts, arms, etc.), we can feel how dense it is; when we grab it, there's substance there. People often misperceive inflammation in the gut for belly fat. When we press on our bellies, it feels more like a marshmallow. I love seeing the reaction on people's faces when I say this, because it's an "aha" moment. That marshmallow isn't belly fat; that's inflammation in the gut from eating foods we are sensitive to. There's a difference. The reason the abdomen "goes down" after avoiding food sensitivities is because we have just reduced the inflammation in the gastrointestinal system and things have had a chance to calm down. This fact usually pulls people in. (Hey, we are all vain sometimes, myself included.) How amazing is it to know we have FULL CONTROL over what we eat and therefore our inflammation levels in the body from what we eat and, as a result of this, we can directly bring down the "puffiness" of our abdomen.

I think we have hammered home the point that food sensitivities cause inflammation. So, what I want to point out to you now is that if there is already an inflammatory condition happening and we are eating foods we are sensitive to, this may serve to piss off said inflammatory condition, which will only result in further discomfort, worse symptoms, more pain, etc. What are some examples of inflammatory conditions? Arthritis, tendonitis, bursitis, some kidney pathologies, and inflammatory bowel disease, just to name a few. Sometimes it takes framing it like this to get people to pay attention to the potential power of avoiding our food sensitivities. Typically when one is living with chronic illness, there can be a sense of helplessness and succumbing to pain and flare-ups. However, realizing the power of food sensitivity avoidance and that what we eat is 100% in OUR control, we are able to TAKE OUR POWER BACK!

The Elimination Diet, also referred to as The Hypoallergenic Diet, is the tool used to uncover which foods we are sensitive to. There are two main phases: elimination and reintroduction. I typically do an initial phase of preparation with my patients so that we can navigate the elimination more successfully. The impact of food sensitivities on health and living in general became a huge thing for me after having my baby. I was like a one-woman army preaching my message to the masses. All I knew was that I needed all the energy I could find and wanted to feel freaking vibrant. I had already gone through the elimination diet more than once at this point and knew what my food sensitivities were and how crappy they made me feel. I avoided those buggers like the plague. Recently someone said to me, as they finished their elimination phase and were feeling so good, that once they found out what the food was that was causing them to feel so shitty, they would run it over with their car! That's the power of food sensitivities.

Back to my story though, it was basically for the sake of my energy and mood and overall just feeling GOOD that I stayed the course in avoiding my food sensitivities postpartum. It wasn't until that one day when I caught a glimpse of myself in the mirror and saw my abdomen that I really went, "Whoa, my stomach is so flat!" It's a nice side effect, I'll admit. HOWEVER, the BEST PART of the whole thing was how COMFORTABLE AND CONFIDENT I began feeling in my own skin. When you feel better in your body approaching your 30s after having a baby than you did when you were a teenager, that is fucking amazing. I reached a point where I realized that I had to tell people about this. It felt selfish and unethical to keep this information to myself. I know that there is a woman reading this right now who has never felt the same in her body since having kids, or who wants that comfortable and confident stance. My love, food sensitivities may be the answer here.

This past summer, I was visiting my aunt, who makes the BEST tiramisu EVER. As I went for it, my dad just said, "It's going to make your stomach hurt" (referring to the gluten). I ate one piece anyway. Then I figured, "Hey, the damage is already done. Hit me with another piece!" (This is a very dangerous thought to have and is bullshit, but hey, we all have our human experiences.) My uncle refilled my plate like any kind host would. Then came the next day. I knew the bloating would be there (it wasn't just gluten, it was the dairy, too), but I also was SO irritable, like super irritable. I was like, "What the heck is this?" Then I realized, "Oh right, the tiramisu." Evidence even supports the theory that inflammation induced from eating foods we are sensitive to can affect mood. Research has found higher levels of inflammatory markers specifically related to gluten food sensitivity in those with major depressive disorder versus healthy controls.[3]

Now, here is the thing. I'm not suggesting that a gluten intolerance is the etiological factor for major depressive disorder, so everyone hold your horses. What I am suggesting is that food sensitivities induce inflammation, and inflammation makes us feel like shit, which can even extend to mood. Are food sensitivities the only thing that affect mood? NO. Are they an intriguing avenue to pursue as a piece of the puzzle when it comes to mood? I would say so. I am all about empowering individuals, and all too often people come to see me in clinic, sit across from me, look me in the eye (or sometimes don't), and profess how out of control they feel or how helpless they feel when it comes to their health. That is NOT a fun place to be. I must take a

---

[3] Hanna Karakula-Juchnowicz et al. "The Food-Specific Serum IgG Reactivity in Major Depressive Disorder Patients, Irritable Bowel Syndrome Patients and Healthy Controls." *Nutrients* 10, no. 5 (2018): 548.

moment here to mention that I honor all of you for taking a step into getting support; you are courageous and inspiring. We can 100% control what we put in our bodies by making the best decisions possible with proper guidance. Avoiding our food sensitivities has the potential to not only make us feel physically better but can even help improve our mood, which is a big deal. We can't control external events, but we sure as hell can control what we feed ourselves (including the bullshit thoughts). Knowing your own food sensitivities gives the power back to you, because you can choose to avoid them and in doing so promote taking control of your own health. You are taking your health into your own hands.

You can't do anything with information you don't have. For a simplified and supportive journey to finding out what YOUR food sensitivities are, you can join me online at: https://drnadia-rizzo-naturopathic-doctor.teachable.com/p/simpleeliminationdiet.

CHAPTER 5: TOXINS, STRESS, AND EXERCISE

What Nobody Tells You About Breaking Down Fat

I know you want to burn that fat, but it is SO important to realize that certain things should be in place first. See, fat stores things. These things get released when the fat breaks down. Makes sense, right? If we have a globule of fat that is holding on to things, when we burn it or bust it open to break it down, the things it was holding on to then release and have to get processed as well. So, if fat is holding on to any toxic waste, we want to make sure we are eliminating it properly. What does this mean? It means your natural routes of elimination need to be supported and functioning well before you go all gung ho breaking down your body fat. The methods of elimination that merit attention include: our bowels, our perspiration, and, of course, our liver.

Let's start with the bowels. You want to have good bowel habits, which means daily movements. You should be able to pass feces without feeling like you are having to push it out, and you want to make sure you're fully evacuating and are actually eliminating everything in there that needs to be eliminated, not just some of it. Our internal plumbing system needs to be intact in order to get rid of the waste that the body wants to eliminate. It's a very clever system, really. Things that I find helpful include proper hydration and using the Squatty Potty ™, which is a stool you place under the toilet to raise your legs and open the colon to improve elimination. Stress can also affect the bowels, and being stressed can make it more difficult to go. Healthy bowels are integral for overall health and are especially important when you break down fat, because you're essentially asking the body to increase its processing of junk elimination.

Next, let's talk about sweat. Listen, sweating is healthy. Perspiration is a method of detox. There is something very important to keep in mind here, ladies, and I am just going to be direct: breasts are literally fat, so when you are trying to break down fat, your boobs might get smaller. (Hey, you are burning fat, right?) So, as this fat burns down and your body releases the junk it has been holding on to, where does it go? You may know this already, but the underarm is an area full of lymph nodes that drain the breast. You want to encourage natural sweating from the area as another means of releasing the junk, and you don't want to clog it with more junk. This means you should stop using antiperspirants in general, particularly those with aluminum. It makes me chuckle when I think of myself as a teenager, going to the gym to sweat it out but using an antiperspirant to literally stop the sweating in my underarm area. Um, hello teenage Nadia! This is one of the most important areas that you want to release the sweat from. Thankfully, I know better now and opt for a more natural deodorant without any antiperspirant action.

Last but not least is your liver. Liver support is super important, but it doesn't have to be extreme. Simple steps like hot lemon water in the morning (which can also help assist with bowel movements) and eliminating alcohol can serve to gently support inherent detox processes.

The Emotional Eating Bit

Whenever I would "stress eat," it usually started with being upset about something, feeling it in my body, and then thinking to myself, "Well Nadia, it's your fault that you are in this situation, so the only person you can be mad at is yourself." I was guilt-tripping myself for a hella long time. The negative self-talk led to the self-sabotage of stress eating, because it's like literally taking out our own internal self-hatred on ourselves. We are mad at ourselves. We are guilt-tripping ourselves. We tell ourselves we should have known or done better. We are punishing ourselves, because we somehow on a subconscious level think it will "even out the score" for what we did. Before I go any further, I want you to get something right the fuck now. You did the best you could with the information you had in the situation you were in at the time. If you keep guilt-tripping yourself, you hold yourself there, and now it's not the other person, the situation, or the external events that hold you down. It's your own damn self.

So, I want you to understand this: YOU MADE NO MISTAKES; you simply had a human experience. We are all spiritual beings having a human experience, not the other way around. Don't forget that every thought you have is heard by your body, and your body listens. What are you instructing it to do? Love the shit out of itself or hate on itself? I am sure you can imagine which will fuel you on your weight loss journey. You need to get to the root of why it's happening, and it all comes back to an emotional source or thought pattern. As I am sure you are beginning to see, weight loss isn't just about diet. It's so much more than that. I always say, "I am more concerned with the words coming out of your mouth than the food going into it."

I highly suggest that you take a moment right now to get onto my free Relentless Self Love Challenge. Click the link to join for free and get seven days of busting through the blocks and breaking the chains that keep you from living the life you truly want to live: http://nadiarizzo.com/relentless-self-love/

Stress Eating Strategy

Before eating, you can ask yourself, "On a scale of 0 to 10, how hungry am I? How stressed am I?" Do a body scan and mindfully tune in to any areas of tension. Start at the top of your head and move down from there, pausing at each body part to check for tension. Is your jaw tense? Is your tongue needing to be returned to the bottom of your mouth and relaxed? Do you feel tightness in your neck, shoulders, or arms? When your attention arrives at the heart area, take a deep breath. What does your gut feel like? Go down to the pelvic area, lower back, hips, thighs, legs, feet, and toes. Check in with yourself. You can even set a daily reminder on your phone that says, "Relax your shoulders." Sometimes we all need the reminder.

Chronic Stress and Why You Need to Skip Going Hardcore at the Gym

When we are stressed out, our adrenal glands (those tiny powerhouses that sit on top of each kidney) pump out cortisol, often referred to as our "stress hormone." This jolt of cortisol helps us to cope with the stressful situation at hand, just like our caveman ancestors who were forced into "fight-or-flight" mode when encountering a potentially life-threatening situation, such as a wild animal hunting them down as prey. So, they could either fight that beast or run the heck outta there. As such, when our body is stressed, the blood shunts to our arms and legs, because we need blood and energy in our arms and legs to help us run away from this animal as fast as possible. When we are literally running for our lives, digesting is not going to save us, so we don't need blood there. This diversion of blood supply away from the digestive system also suppresses bowel movements (because that's definitely not going to help you in an emergency situation).

The point here is we are built to handle this short-term jolt of stress, because we have survival instincts in us still. However, welcome to the second millennium where the majority of us reading this book, I am assuming, are not running for our lives from a wild animal. Yet, we still experience fight-or-flight when we get into an argument with a loved one, have deadlines to meet, find ourselves in a traffic jam, go through a divorce, and experience financial troubles. The source of the stress is different, but the body responds the same way. Another major difference between us and our cavemen ancestors is that their stress was truly in the moment, running for their lives. Our stress is long term these days, and this, my friends, we were not made to naturally deal with, especially not without proper management. Long-term stress can wreak havoc on the body and mind. When we are in an acute situation, our adrenal glands pump out a burst of cortisol to help us deal and get through it. But when we are in a chronic state of stress, after a while our adrenal glands start to get worn out, and instead of compensating with additional cortisol, they start to get fatigued and can actually begin to produce less cortisol. This is what is referred to as "adrenal fatigue." Long-term stress can literally burn out our poor powerhouse adrenals, and this is a strike against us when it comes to weight loss.

Now, just as the body responds the same way when we are agitated in a traffic jam as it did when our cavemen ancestors were running from wild animals, the body responds the same way to stress, regardless of the reason we are stressed. Whether we are planning a fun and exciting (yet still stressful) wedding or we are going through long-term job loss and financial stress, the body responds the same way. It doesn't matter whether it's "good" or "bad" stress; the body just sees it as stress and has the same response. For someone who is dealing with adrenal fatigue, any additional stress is like beating the system when it is already down and compromised. So, how does this relate to exercise? If we are doing INTENSE exercise, like really pounding it out, and we have adrenal fatigue, we are beating down a system that is already knocked down. See how this isn't a great idea? Now, again, I am talking about a person who actually has adrenal fatigue, not a healthy individual with managed stress and no compromise in natural cortisol production. And I am definitely not knocking exercising. It's just that so many of us have long-term stress that doesn't go properly managed and who probably didn't even know about adrenal fatigue or never had it explained to them.

If you are wondering if you have adrenal fatigue, see your board-certified, licensed Naturopathic Doctor for proper lab work and assessment. If you have adrenal fatigue and are trying to lose weight, it's important to avoid intense exercise and to practice gentle activities such as yoga, Pilates, and moderately paced walking.

CHAPTER 6:
THE BIGGER PICTURE

I love you, I honor you, and I am so grateful for you.

This has been the first chunk of time I've been single since I was 17 years old. We're talking two fiancés and an adorable love of my life, my heart and soul munchkin later. During the first year of my separation, I retreated into a bubble of deep self-healing and reflection. The most physically attractive man could've walked by and I would not have even noticed. I didn't even own makeup until I had scheduled Christmas pictures with my son and figured a little foundation couldn't hurt. Today, I learned an important lesson in discernment. I found myself in a situation where I could spend my day with one of two men, and neither one felt right. One was a guy who seemed nice enough in our brief messaging, but when I saw him in person, I just got jerk vibes. Then, of course, the night before an "old friend/

short flame" had messaged me to see if I wanted to meet up the next day. (This is the same one I mentioned in the beginning—you know, the gummy bears down the hatch after officially "parting ways.") All I'm sensing from them is that it's so not aligned and not where I am meant to be. So, I am faced with a choice: meet up with one of them anyway to kill time since there's nothing else going on tonight, or pass it up and honor myself by choosing to spend my time only doing what I intuitively know is aligned with what is right for me. I ended up taking myself out for a bite and a (virgin) drink. I even wore the red dress, heels, and sat at the bar area. It felt so fucking good. Why am I telling you all this? Because sometimes we need a reminder that we can treat ourselves like queens. You know how they say, "What's a queen without her king?" Well, I say, "She's still a motherfucking queen. Rock that crown, baby."

It's now been over a year that I've been on my own, and it's been an amazing journey inward and a huge self-love adventure. One thing I have definitely learned and experienced, not just simply read in books, is that you really do need to honor and love yourself. How you want someone else to treat you is how you need to be treating yourself. That includes how you speak to yourself, how you take yourself out, and how you respect yourself. **Taking care of yourself is a form of self-love and self-respect.** Why am I including this in a weight loss book? Because every single cell in your body listens to every thought you have, even the silent ones, even the ones you wouldn't dare say aloud. Every single cell in your body responds to how you treat yourself, and you know what, the universe responds to that, too. The way you treat yourself is like saying, "This is the standard I set, and this is what I am ok with." And then, guess what? The universe responds by matching what you are putting out and brings you more of exactly that. Then you complain about being in the same place and wondering why this shit keeps happening to you. Change your vibrational frequency by changing your habits and your self-talk. Look in the mirror and say, "I love you. You are so sexy, you are so beautiful, you are so amazing, and I honor you and I forgive you." Just do it, every day, even on the days when you're not sure you believe it. You will begin to **embody that energy.** Watch how different your life becomes.

Start Where You Are

We all have either been or know that person who does things full-on, gung ho, 180-degree-turn style. How well did that work out? Even if it did work out at first, how long did that last for? I can promise you, not long. Listen, you need to meet yourself where you are. This journey is one step at a time. One change that is implemented as a habit for three weeks and more is going to serve you better than two weeks of full-on change followed by forever falling off the bandwagon. Changing your life one step at a time helps that change to be sustainable long term. This isn't a "diet program." This is YOUR LIFE. And these principles can be applied to any area of life, not just nutrition and health.

For example, I have recently started reading an amazing financial advising book. *Smart Women Finish Rich* by David

Bach, who is a financial expert and amazing mentor to so many women. I started doing the steps of this program by making one simple change: putting 10% of all gross (not net) income into a savings account. Then I cut up one of my credit cards. I didn't just hide it; I actually chopped it into bits and tossed the remnants. Everything was going smoothly until one day I was reading the book, standing by the coffee bar at my brother's house while my son slept nearby. It was the chapter about future financial planning, wills, and living trusts. "Ok," I thought to myself, "I have to set up a living trust." But that felt way too overwhelming in that moment. So, I made a note in my calendar to contact a lawyer and set up an appointment to get these documents sorted for a living trust in one month. I literally had to shut the book and step away. I realized I still had much of the book left to read and wondered what the hell else this guy was going to have me do in the pages to follow. I had to meet myself where I was, so I decided it was ok to continue with the good habits I had already begun to implement, to set a goal of tackling the living trust in a month, and to set the book aside for now.

See, here's the thing. Had I tried to do it all at once, I would just have gotten overwhelmed and would have fallen off the bandwagon. In these cases when we feel overloaded and then we feel like, "Oh man, I should be doing these 10 other things and I'm not doing them yet. I'm so behind!," we feel defeated. It makes us feel like shit, which doesn't help us improve. With my finances, I was still **showing up and doing the steps I had committed to regularly, keeping those habits, and then setting a deadline for the next step.** I knew I couldn't read further until the next step was implemented, because I didn't want to get overloaded. My commitment and showing up to the already-implemented steps **gave me a sense of accomplishment.** It is this sense of accomplishment that kept me going and gave me the confidence that I could take the next steps and be successful at them. I didn't leave them open-ended. I set an exact deadline, and I intend to keep it.

Don't get overloaded. Take one step at a time. It takes three weeks for a behavior to be formed as a habit. Once you have the first step down, then add step two. I do exactly this with many of my patients in private practice. We agree on what we would like to accomplish long term, and then we start with ONE change. I cannot tell you how many times I have seen the relief on people's faces when they realize I am not going to try to force them to change 100 things overnight. This isn't a race. It's your health, and it's your life. It is much better to **get there the right way and to stay there** than try to change everything at once and never get there at all.

Knowing Your Why

Before you even tell me the details of your goal and your timeline and how you want it to happen (spoiler alert: you need to drop the how—more on this soon), I want to know your **why.** When you say to me that you want to lose weight, I want to know why. When you say to me it is so you can fit into size whatever jeans, I want to know why. When you say it's because you want to feel attractive to someone else, I want to know why. I want to know what the worst-case scenario is that you have thought up in your mind if this doesn't happen. If you don't lose the weight, what would that mean? If it doesn't happen, what is the worst possible thing that could be true as a result of that?

FYI, I am super passionate about this bit and haven't hit the keys on my keyboard this hard the entire time I've been writing this book. I feel angry, frustrated, and fired up, because we think up so much false shit in our minds that take us down a very unnecessary, made-up path. We can believe whatever we want to. The minute we truly realize that we are in control of our own thoughts and subjective experience, that is the minute our life will completely change for the better. You control your thoughts. Your thoughts carry energetic vibrations and become your beliefs. Your beliefs become your entire life, including your body. The worst thing you could ever do is talk to yourself like you don't love yourself or believe you aren't worthy of having something. You are worthy of all of your highest desires simply because God put you into existence. If you don't realize that is enough, then nothing will ever be enough.

Your why is what keeps you going. Your why is beneath it all. Wanting to fit into a certain size or feel attractive to someone or have amazing sex isn't about all of those things deep down.

Those are just the surface expressions of something deeper. Let's play out a little example of this:

Dr. Nadia: *What is your goal?*

Sandra: *To lose 50 pounds.*

Chapter 6: The Bigger Picture

Dr. Nadia: *Why do you want to lose 50 pounds?*

Sandra: *So I can fit into smaller clothes, have more energy, and feel better.*

Dr. Nadia: *What do you mean by "feel better"?*

Sandra: *I just don't want to carry around all this extra weight. It's exhausting. I can't do things I used to do and I am tired of it.*

Dr. Nadia: *Well, what is it you want to do exactly?*

Sandra: *Play with my grandkids.*

Dr. Nadia: *Ok, well you still do things together that are sedentary, like painting, doing arts and crafts, and playing music.*

Sandra: *Yes, but I want to run with them. My granddaughter loves playing at the park, and I can barely keep up with her. I can't even stand and move around for long periods of time baking with her or playing catch with my grandson. I feel like a boring old grandma.*

Dr. Nadia: *And what does this mean to feel like a boring old grandma?*

Sandra: *It means I don't do things they want to do, or I can't do things they want to do.*

Dr. Nadia: *So, what is the worst thing that can happen if you are never doing things that your grandkids want to do and only doing other activities, like going to the cinema to watch a film?*

Sandra: *If I can't do things they want to do, they will look back on memories of our time together and think of how boring I was because I couldn't interact with them in the fun ways they wanted me to. And then they won't even want to spend time with me.*

Dr. Nadia: *So, it sounds like why you are really here is because you want to have amazing times with your grandkids—times that they can look back on and cherish forever, memories that make them feel good when they think of you.*

Sandra; *Yes, exactly. That's exactly why I'm here.*

Dr. Nadia: *Great! Now that we have that straight, we can move forward.*

Do you get it? If all Sandra were to tell herself is that she wants to lose 50 pounds, it's kind of like whatever, or vague, or disconnected. It's abstract. When we connect with her *why*, we hit the emotion and actually get to the heart. If every day Sandra tells herself, "I get to spend time with my grandkids and make amazing memories that they will cherish forever," that is what will keep her going. It will keep her going on the days when she has had enough and she is questioning it all, and it will actually motivate her to stick to it. The why isn't the skinny jeans; heck, it's not even the 50 pounds. The why is what it means deep down. Usually if we ask ourselves, "What is the worst thing that could happen if I don't accomplish x," we get to the why. **Freaking know your why.**

Do this exercise, and pretend I am there with you. Do NOT stop until you get to your true why. You will know exactly when it happens when you uncover it. Even if you think you know your why, do this exercise anyway. You might be surprised by what you learn. I've done it with many other goals in my life, too. Take your why, write it on a piece of paper, stick it up on your bathroom mirror or bedside table, and set a daily reminder on your phone as reinforcement. So, for Sandra, it would be, "I make amazing memories with my grandkids that they cherish forever when they think of me." Phrase it positively. Don't write what you don't want; only write what you are manifesting, what you do desire. The constant exposure to this—when you wake up in the morning, as you go about your day, and before you go to sleep at night—will embed it into your subconscious and into reality. There is so much power to this, so use it only for good intentions.

You don't want to risk the universe just taking your bad intentions and boomeranging them back to you. I can't stress this enough: only write down the positive desired outcome. That is the vibration we are manifesting, and the good outcome being reality.

Belief and Visualization… Because It Already Is as Such

Ok, now this might seem a bit "woo woo" but, hey, you are here because you need to hear all of this, and I won't leave you without every tool I can possibly put within these pages. Visualization is an extremely powerful tool. Manifestation coaches in various fields talk about this all of the time. What you need to know is that visualization alone is missing a key component: the feeling. When we visualize the outcome we want, it is also important to think about what that would feel like. What does it feel like to be in that state, already having accomplished that goal, having that whatever? Sit with that feeling. Really sit with it. This doesn't have to be time-consuming, just a few minutes a day will do. I've done this so many times while writing this book. I know this book will help millions. I have even titled my Google Docs folder of this manuscript: "I help millions with this book." Before sitting down to type tonight, I thought about what it is going to feel like being on TV to share this information on a show I know I will be on. I felt the love, the excitement, the warmth, the joy, all of it. I am freaking excited. I hold onto that feeling, I feel it, I sit with it, and every time I picture this final product—the book with its cover, all set, in my hands, your hands, and the hands of my millions of readers over time—I know it is reality (and obviously so because you are reading these words right now!).

So, let me remind you: sexy isn't a number. It's not your dress size, how tall you are, how small your waist is, or how big your boobs are. "Sexiness" is not something you create. It is something you tap into. You are the most attractive to yourself, others, and all good energies when you are living in alignment with your true nature. **We are spiritual beings having a human experience,** not the other way around. Our true nature is light, with high vibrational frequency. We are the most attracted to those around us who are in touch with their spirit, who are living in their light because it reminds us of who we really are and that is truly what we want to return to. We are the most attractive when we are shedding ourselves, not of the pounds, but of the negativity, the guilt, and any low vibrational state. The *body* hears every thought we have and responds. The *universe* hears every thought we have and responds. If there is one thing to do in order to be sexy, it is to live in your light, to find your soul's mission, and to live every day to accomplish that mission. The body will respond. When we are solely doing it from a physical plane of operation—that is, doing the diet and exercise but neglecting the soul and the mind—the results are not sustainable; they're only temporary. When we are living in our light, we are making a permanent change and reminding others that they can do the same. For even just a moment, when we come into contact with another being vibrating at that high frequency of our true nature, we spark a remembrance of the soul, a remembrance of who we really are and what we came here to do. And there is nothing sexier than that.

ACKNOWLEDGMENTS

I acknowledge that I am only a vessel who has agreed to transmit the soul and heartfelt messages within these pages. I acknowledge a divine power that is far greater than me, one that I am never separated from, and one that is always calling me back to a place of remembrance of my true nature, grace, and love.

I'd like to thank my son for always fueling me to be the best possible version of myself I can be.

I thank my parents and brother for always being there for me, regardless of the circumstances, and supporting me in every possible way.

I thank my friends & family at large for the love and support during the struggles and for the many laughs and consistent heartfelt times.

I thank my dear friend, Peter Aroukatos, who always seems to know exactly what to say to make me laugh, make me feel better, and help steer me in the right direction.

I thank my dear friend and colleague, Dr. Laura Belus, who was my accountability partner throughout this journey and was constantly pushing me to get this work out into the world.

I thank the men I have loved, for each have helped me grow to spiritual heights and experience the human events needed to learn the lessons, deepen my own self-love, and continue on learning.

I thank all of my mentors and coaches and all of the lightworkers and spiritual teachers who are serving from a place of love and who have shared their message with me and the world.

I thank each and every one of you, readers, for being here, for sharing this space with me, and for allowing me to be a part of your journey. I honor each and every one of you.

CPSIA information can be obtained
at www.ICGtesting.com
Printed in the USA
BVHW040435090121
597434BV00002B/6